PLANT BASED DIET

COOKBOOK FOR WOMAN

2021

50 Amazing and Mouth-watering recipes to lose weight and prevent diabetes. Lose weight fast with fast and mouth-watering recipes for everyday meals.

Ursa Males

TABLE OF CONTENTS

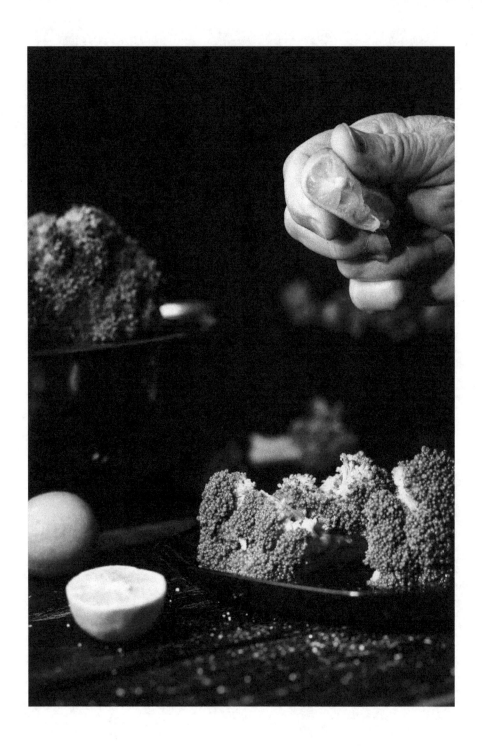

BREAKFAST

1. Sunshine Muffins

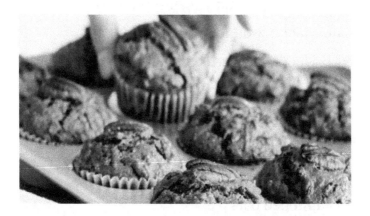

Preparation time: 15 minutes

Cooking time: 30 minutes

Servings: 6

Ingredients:

- 1 teaspoon coconut oil for greasing muffin tins (optional)
- 2 tablespoons almond butter/sunflower seed butter
- ¼ cup non-dairy milk
- 1 orange, peeled
- 1 carrot, coarsely chopped
- 2 tablespoons chopped dried apricots/other dried fruit
- 3 tablespoons molasses

- 2 tablespoons ground flaxseed
- 1 teaspoon apple cider vinegar
- 1 teaspoon pure vanilla extract
- ½ teaspoon ground cinnamon
- ½ teaspoon ground ginger (optional)
- ¼ teaspoon ground nutmeg (optional)
- ¼ teaspoon allspice (optional)
- ¾ cup rolled oats or whole-grain flour
- 1 teaspoon baking powder
- ½ teaspoon baking soda
- Mix-ins (optional):
- ½ cup rolled oats
- 2 tablespoons raisins or other chopped dried fruit
- 2 tablespoons sunflower seeds

Directions:

1. Preheat the oven to 350°F. Prepare a 6-cup muffin tin by rubbing the cups' insides with coconut oil or using silicone or paper muffin cups.
2. Purée the nut butter, milk, orange, carrot, apricots, molasses, flaxseed, vinegar, vanilla, cinnamon, ginger, nutmeg, and allspice in a food processor or blender until somewhat smooth.
3. Grind the oats in a clean coffee grinder until they're consistent with flour (or use whole-grain flour). In a

large bowl, mix the oats with the baking powder and baking soda.

4. Mix the wet ingredients into the dry ingredients until just combined. Fold in the mix-ins (if using).
5. Spoon about ¼ cup batter into each muffin cup and bake for 30 minutes, or until a toothpick inserted into the center comes out clean.

Nutrition: Calories: 287 Fat: 12g Carbs: 41g Protein: 8g

2. Applesauce Crumble Muffins

Preparation time: 15 minutes

Cooking time: 15-20 minutes

Servings: 12

Ingredients:

- 1 teaspoon coconut oil for greasing muffin tins (optional)
- 2 tablespoons nut butter or seed butter
- 1½ cups unsweetened applesauce
- 1/3 cup coconut sugar
- ½ cup non-dairy milk
- 2 tablespoons ground flaxseed
- 1 teaspoon apple cider vinegar
- 1 teaspoon pure vanilla extract
- 2 cups whole-grain flour
- 1 teaspoon baking soda
- ½ teaspoon baking powder
- 1 teaspoon ground cinnamon
- Pinch sea salt
- ½ cup walnuts, chopped
- Toppings (optional):
- ¼ cup walnuts

- ¼ cup of coconut sugar
- ½ teaspoon ground cinnamon

Directions:

1. Preheat the oven to 350°F. Prepare two 6-cup muffin tins by rubbing the cups' insides with coconut oil or using silicone or paper muffin cups.
2. In a large bowl, mix the nut butter, applesauce, coconut sugar, milk, flaxseed, vinegar, and vanilla until thoroughly combined, or purée in a food processor or blender.
3. In another large bowl, sift together the flour, baking soda, baking powder, cinnamon, salt, and chopped walnuts. Mix the dry ingredients into the wet ingredients until just combined.
4. Spoon about ¼ cup batter into each muffin cup and sprinkle with the topping of your choice (if using). Bake for 15 to 20 minutes, or until a toothpick inserted into the center comes out clean.

Nutrition: Calories: 287 Fat: 12g Carbs: 41g Protein: 8g

3. Baked Banana French Toast with Raspberry Syrup

Preparation time: 10 minutes

Cooking time: 30 minutes

Servings: 8 slices

Ingredients:

- For the French toast:
- 1 banana
- 1 cup of coconut milk
- 1 teaspoon pure vanilla extract
- ¼ teaspoon ground nutmeg
- ½ teaspoon ground cinnamon
- 1½ teaspoons arrowroot powder or flour
- Pinch sea salt
- 8 slices whole-grain bread
- For the raspberry syrup:
- 1 cup raspberries/other berries
- 2 tablespoons water, or pure fruit juice
- 1 to 2 tablespoons maple syrup or coconut sugar (optional)

Directions:

1. For the French toast, preheat the oven to 350°F. In a shallow bowl, purée or mash the banana well. Mix in the coconut milk, vanilla, nutmeg, cinnamon, arrowroot, and salt.

2. Dip the slices of bread in the banana mixture, and then lay them out in a 13-by-9-inch baking dish. They should cover the bottom of the dish and overlap slightly but shouldn't be stacked on top of each other.

3. Pour any leftover banana mixture over the bread, and put the dish in the oven—Bake within 30 minutes, or until the tops are lightly browned. Serve topped with raspberry syrup.

4. To Make the Raspberry Syrup:

5. Heat the raspberries in a small pot with the water and the maple syrup (if using) on medium heat.

6. Leave to simmer, stirring occasionally, and breaking up the berries for 15 to 20 minutes, until the liquid has reduced.

Nutrition: Calories: 166 Fat: 7g Carbs: 23g Protein: 5g

4. Cinnamon Apple Toast

Preparation time: 5 minutes

Cooking time: 10-20 minutes

Servings: 12

Ingredients:

- 1 to 2 teaspoons coconut oil
- ½ teaspoon ground cinnamon
- 1 tablespoon maple syrup or coconut sugar
- 1 apple, cored and thinly sliced
- 2 slices whole-grain bread

Directions:

1. In a large bowl, mix the coconut oil, cinnamon, and maple syrup. Add the apple slices and toss with your hands to coat them.
2. To panfry the toast, place the apple slices in a medium skillet on medium-high and cook for about 5 minutes, or until slightly soft, then transfer to a plate.
3. Cook the bread in the same skillet for 2 to 3 minutes on each side. Top the toast with the apples. Alternately, you can bake the toast.

4. Use your hands to rub each slice of bread with some of the coconut oil mixtures on both sides. Lay them on a small baking sheet, top with the coated apples.

Nutrition: Calories: 187 Fat: 8g Carbs: 27g Protein: 4g

5. **Muesli and Berries Bowl**

Preparation time: 10 minutes

Cooking time: 0 minutes

Servings: 5

Ingredients:

- For the muesli:
- 1 cup rolled oats
- 1 cup spelt flakes, or quinoa flakes, or more rolled oats
- 2 cups puffed cereal
- ¼ cup sunflower seeds
- ¼ cup almonds
- ¼ cup raisins
- ¼ cup dried cranberries
- ¼ cup chopped dried figs
- ¼ cup unsweetened shredded coconut
- ¼ cup non-dairy chocolate chips
- 1 to 3 teaspoons ground cinnamon
- For the bowl:
- ½ cup non-dairy milk, or unsweetened applesauce
- ¾ cup muesli
- ½ cup berries

Directions:

1. Put the muesli ingredients in a container or bag and shake. Combine the muesli and bowl ingredients in a bowl or to-go container.

Nutrition: Calories: 441 Fat: 20g Carbs: 63g Protein: 10g

6. Chocolate Quinoa Breakfast Bowl

Preparation time: 5 minutes

Cooking time: 30 minutes

Servings: 2

Ingredients:

- 1 cup quinoa
- 1 teaspoon ground cinnamon
- 1 cup non-dairy milk
- 1 cup of water
- 1 large banana
- 2 to 3 tablespoons unsweetened cocoa powder or carob
- 1 to 2 tablespoons almond butter or other nut or seed butter
- 1 tablespoon ground flaxseed, or chia or hemp seeds
- 2 tablespoons walnuts
- ¼ cup raspberries

Directions:

1. Put the quinoa, cinnamon, milk, and water in a medium pot. Bring to a boil over high heat, then turn down low and simmer, covered, for 25 to 30 minutes.
2. While the quinoa is simmering, purée or mash the banana in a medium bowl and stir in the cocoa powder, almond butter, and flaxseed.

3. To serve, spoon 1 cup cooked quinoa into a bowl, top with half the pudding and half the walnuts and raspberries.

Nutrition: Calories: 392 Fat: 19g Carbs: 49g Protein: 12g

7. Fruit Salad with Zesty Citrus Couscous

Preparation time: 5 minutes

Cooking time: 5 minutes

Servings: 1

Ingredients:

- 1 orange, zested, and juiced
- ¼ cup whole-wheat couscous, or corn couscous
- 1 cup assorted berries (strawberries, blackberries, blueberries)
- ½ cup cubed or balled melon (cantaloupe or honeydew)
- 1 tablespoon maple syrup or coconut sugar (optional)
- 1 tablespoon fresh mint, minced (optional)
- 1 tablespoon unsweetened coconut flakes

Directions:

1. Put the orange juice in a small pot, add half the zest, and bring to a boil. Put the dry couscous in a small bowl and pour the boiling orange juice over it.

2. If there isn't enough juice to fully submerge the couscous, add just enough boiling water to do so. Cover the bowl with a plate or seal with wrap, and let steep for 5 minutes.

3. In a medium bowl, toss the berries and melon with the maple syrup (if using) and the rest of the zest. You can either keep the fruit cool or heat it lightly in the small pot you used for the orange juice.

4. When the couscous is soft, remove the cover and fluff it with a fork. Top with fruit, fresh mint, and coconut.

Nutrition: Calories: 496 Fat: 10g Carbs: 97g Protein: 11g

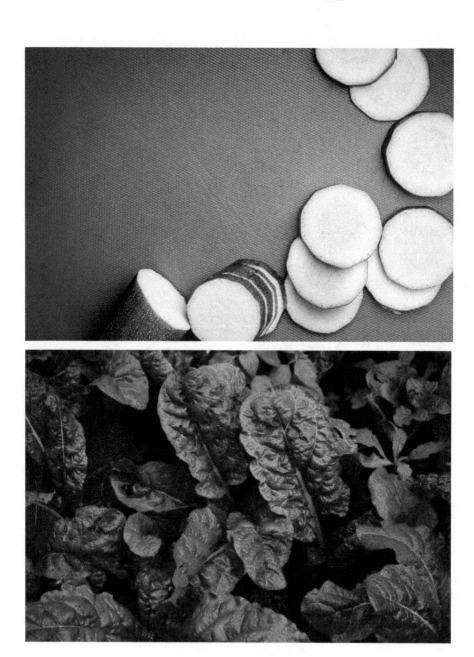

LUNCH

8. Chickpea Salad Bites

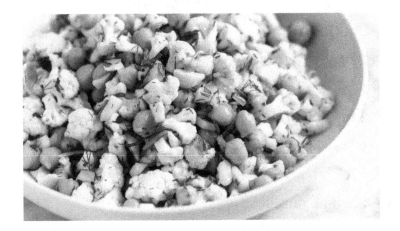

Preparation time: 15 minutes

Cooking time: 0 minutes

Servings: 4

Ingredients:

- For the Bread:
- 2 tablespoons chopped parsley
- 1 small green chili pepper
- 1/3 cup of raisins
- 1 teaspoon garlic powder
- ½ teaspoon salt
- 1/3 teaspoon ground black pepper

- ½ teaspoon smoked paprika
- ½ tablespoon maple syrup
- ½ teaspoon cayenne pepper
- 2 tablespoons balsamic vinegar
- 1 1/2 cups crumbled rye bread, whole-grain
- For the Salad:
- 2 scallions, chopped
- 1/3 cup chopped pickles
- 2 tablespoons chopped chives and more for topping
- ½ teaspoon minced garlic
- 1 ½ cup cooked chickpeas
- 1 lemon, juiced
- ½ teaspoon salt
- ¼ teaspoon ground black pepper
- 1 tablespoon poppy seed
- 1 teaspoon mustard paste
- 1/3 cup coconut yogurt

Directions:

1. Prepare the bread, and for this, place all of its ingredients in a food processor and then pulse for 1 minute until just combined; don't overmix.
2. Then make bites of the bread mixture and for this, take a 2.3-inch round cookie cutter, add 2 tablespoons of the bread mixture, press it into the cutter, and gently

lift it out; repeat with the remaining batter to make seven more bites.

3. Prepare the salad and for this, take a large bowl, add chickpeas in it, then add chives, scallion, pickles, and garlic, and then mash chickpeas by using a fork until broken.

4. Add remaining ingredients for the salad and stir until well mixed. Assemble the bites and for this, top each prepared bread bite generously with prepared salad, sprinkle with chives and poppy seeds, and then serve.

Nutrition: Cal 210 Fat 4 g Carbohydrates 36 g Protein 7 g

9. Avocado and Chickpeas Lettuce Cups

Preparation time: 10 minutes

Cooking time: 0 minutes

Servings: 4

Ingredients:

- 2 small avocados, peeled, pitted, diced
- 8 ounces hearts of palm
- ¾ cup cooked chickpeas
- 1/2 cup cucumber, diced
- 1 tablespoon minced shallots
- 2 cups mixed greens
- 1 tablespoon Dijon mustard
- 1 lime, zested, juiced
- 2 tablespoons chopped cilantro and more for topping
- 2/3 teaspoon salt
- 1/3 teaspoon ground black pepper
- 1 tablespoon apple cider vinegar
- 2 ½ tablespoons olive oil

Directions:

1. Take a medium bowl, add shallots and cilantro in it, stir in salt, black pepper, mustard, vinegar, lime juice, and zest until just mixed, and then slowly mix in olive oil until combined.

2. Add cucumber, hearts of palm, and chickpeas, stir until mixed, fold in avocado and then top with some more cilantro.

3. Distribute mixed greens among four plates, top with chickpea mixture, and then serve.

Nutrition: Cal 280 Fat 12.6 g Carbohydrates 32.8 g Protein 7.6 g

10. **Pesto Quinoa with White Beans**

Preparation time: 5 minutes

Cooking time: 15 minutes

Servings: 4

Ingredients:

- 12 ounces cooked white bean
- 3 ½ cups quinoa, cooked
- 1 medium zucchini, sliced
- ¾ cup sun-dried tomato
- ¼ cup pine nuts
- 1 tablespoon olive oil
- For the Pesto:
- 1/3 cup walnuts
- 2 cups arugula
- 1 teaspoon minced garlic
- 2 cups basil
- ¾ teaspoon salt
- ¼ teaspoon ground black pepper
- 1 tablespoon lemon juice
- 1/3 cup olive oil
- 2 tablespoons water

Directions:

1. Prepare the pesto, place all of its ingredients in a food processor and pulse for 2 minutes until smooth, scraping the sides of the container frequently, and set aside until required.

2. Take a large skillet pan, place it over medium heat, add oil and when hot, add zucchini and cook for 4 minutes until tender-crisp.

3. Season zucchini with salt and black pepper, cook for 2 minutes until lightly brown, add tomatoes and white beans and continue cooking for 4 minutes until white beans begin to crisp.

4. Stir in pine nuts, cook for 2 minutes until toasted, remove the pan from heat, and transfer the zucchini mixture into a medium bowl.

5. Add quinoa and pesto, stir until well combined, then distribute among four bowls and then serve.

Nutrition: Cal 352 Fat 27.3 g Carbohydrates 33.7 g Protein 9.7 g

11. **Pumpkin Risotto**

Preparation time: 5 minutes

Cooking time: 20 minutes

Servings: 4

Ingredients:

- 1 cup Arborio rice
- ½ cup cooked and chopped pumpkin
- 1/2 cup mushrooms
- 1 rib of celery, diced
- ½ of a medium white onion, peeled, diced
- ½ teaspoon minced garlic
- ½ teaspoon salt
- 1/3 teaspoon ground black pepper
- 1 tablespoon olive oil
- ½ tablespoon coconut butter
- 1 cup pumpkin puree
- 2 cups vegetable stock

Directions:

1. Take a medium saucepan, place it over medium heat, add oil, and when hot, add onion and celery, stir in garlic, and cook for 3 minutes until onions begin to soften.

2. Put mushrooms, flavor with salt and black pepper, and cook for 5 minutes.

3. Add rice, pour in pumpkin puree, then gradually pour in the stock until rice soaked up all the liquid and have turned soft.

4. Add butter, remove the pan from heat, stir until creamy mixture comes together, and then serve.

Nutrition: Cal 218.5 Fat 5.2 g Carbohydrates 32.3 g Protein 6.3 g

12. __Garlic Mozzarella Bread__

Preparation time: 15 minutes

Cooking time: 50 minutes

Servings: 8

Ingredients:

- 1 cup mozzarella
- 1 cup almond flour
- ½ medium onion (diced)
- 4 tbsp. ground flaxseed
- 3 tbsp. olive oil
- ½ cup of water
- 1 tbsp. Italian herbs
- ½ tsp. baking powder
- 2 garlic cloves (minced)
- Optional: ¼ cup black olives

Directions:

1. Warm oven to 350°F/175°C and lines a large loaf pan with parchment paper.
2. Combine the water with the ground flaxseed in a small bowl. Let the flaxseed soak for about 10 minutes.
3. Put the soaked seeds in a food processor with all the other ingredients, and pulse until they are combined into a smooth batter.

4. Transfer the batter onto the loaf pan and let the mixture sit for a few minutes. Put the loaf pan in the oven and bake the bread for 50 minutes, until the bread is firm and browned on top.

5. Remove the loaf pan out of the oven and allow the bread to cool down completely. Move the bread to your cutting board, then slice it into 8 slices. Serve and enjoy!

Nutrition: Calories: 256 Carbs: 4.2 g Fat: 23.5 g Protein: 6.6 g

13. __Truffle Parmesan Bread__

Preparation time: 15 minutes

Cooking time: 50 minutes

Servings: 8

Ingredients:

- 1 cup truffle parmesan cheese
- 1 cup almond flour
- ½ cup button mushrooms (diced)
- 2 tbsp. soy sauce
- ½ medium onion (finely chopped)
- ½ cup ground flaxseed
- 4 tbsp. olive oil
- ½ cup of water
- 1 tsp. dried thyme
- 1 tsp. dried basil
- 1 tsp. black pepper
- ½ tsp. baking powder

Directions:

1. Warm oven to 350°F/175°C and lines a large loaf pan with parchment paper.
2. Combine the water with the ground flaxseed in a small bowl. Let the flaxseed soak for about 10 minutes.

3. Meanwhile, put a medium-sized frying pan over medium-high heat and add a tablespoon of olive oil.

4. When the oil is warm, add the chopped onions, mushrooms, and soy sauce to the frying pan and stir-fry until the mushrooms and onion have softened.

5. Put the flaxseed, stir-fried ingredients, and all remaining ingredients in a food processor and pulse until all ingredients are combined into a smooth mixture.

6. Put the batter into your loaf pan and let the mixture sit for a few minutes.

7. Put the loaf pan in the oven and bake the bread for about 50 minutes, until the bread is firm and browned on top. Remove the loaf pan out of the oven and allow the bread to cool down completely.

8. Move the bread to your cutting board, then slice it into 8 slices. Serve warm or cold and enjoy!

Nutrition: Calories: 296 Carbs: 5 g. Fat: 26.9 g. Protein: 7.7 g.

14. **Truffle Parmesan Salad**

Preparation time: 15 minutes

Cooking time: 0 minutes

Servings: 4

Ingredients:

- 4 cups kale (chopped)
- ½ cup truffle parmesan cheese
- 1 tsp. Dijon mustard
- 2 tbsp. olive oil
- 2 tbsp. lemon juice
- Salt and pepper to taste
- Optional: 2 tbsp. water

Directions:

1. Rinse the kale with cold water, then drain the kale and put it into a large bowl. In a medium-sized bowl, mix the remaining ingredients into a dressing. Pour the dressing over the kale and stir gently to cover the kale evenly.

2. Transfer the large bowl to the fridge and allow the salad to chill for up to one hour – doing so will guarantee a better flavor.

3. Alternatively, the salad can be served right away. Enjoy!

Nutrition: Calories: 199 Carbs: 8.5 g. Fat: 16.6 g. Protein: 3.5 g.

15. Cashew Siam Salad

Preparation time: 15 minutes

Cooking time: 0 minutes

Servings: 4

Ingredients:

- Salad:
- 4 cups baby spinach (rinsed, drained)
- ½ cup pickled red cabbage
- Dressing:
- 1-inch piece ginger (finely chopped)
- 1 tsp. chili garlic paste
- 1 tbsp. soy sauce
- ½ tbsp. rice vinegar
- 1 tbsp. sesame oil
- 3 tbsp. avocado oil
- Toppings:
- ½ cup raw cashews (unsalted)
- Optional: ¼ cup fresh cilantro (chopped)

Directions:

1. Put the spinach and red cabbage in a large bowl. Toss to combine and set the salad aside.
2. Toast the cashews in a frying pan over medium-high heat, occasionally stirring until the cashews are golden

brown. It should take about 3 minutes. Turn off the heat and set the frying pan aside.

3. Mix all the dressing ingredients in a medium-sized bowl and use a spoon to mix them into a smooth dressing. Pour the dressing over the spinach salad and top with the toasted cashews.

4. Toss the salad to combine all ingredients and transfer the large bowl to the fridge. Let the salad to chill for up to one hour – doing so will guarantee a better flavor.

5. Alternatively, the salad can be served right away, topped with the optional cilantro. Enjoy!

Nutrition: Calories: 236 Carbs: 6.1 g. Fat: 21.6 g. Protein: 4.2 g.

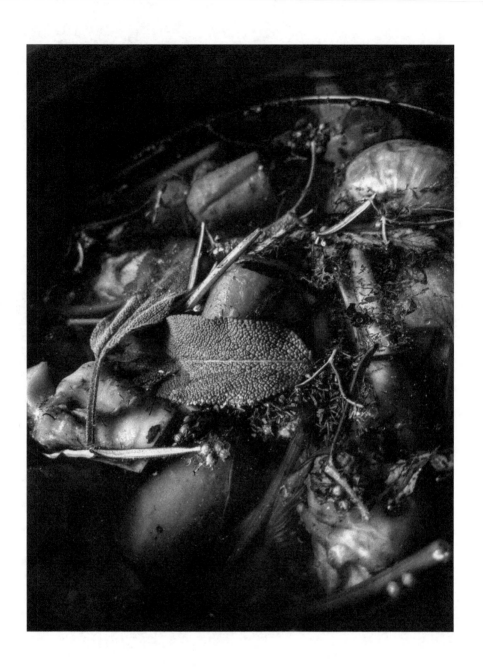

DINNER

16.   <u>**Broccoli & Black Beans Stir Fry**</u>

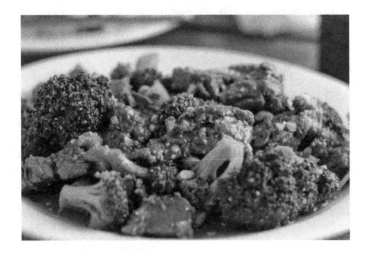

Preparation time: 15 minutes

Cooking time: 10 minutes

Servings: 6

Ingredients:

- 4 cups broccoli florets
- 2 cups cooked black beans
- 1 tablespoon sesame oil
- 4 teaspoons sesame seeds
- 2 cloves garlic, finely minced
- 2 teaspoons ginger, finely chopped
- A large pinch red chili flake

- A pinch turmeric powders
- Salt to taste
- Lime juice to taste (optional)

Directions:

1. Steam broccoli for 6 minutes. Drain and set aside. Warm the sesame oil in your large frying pan over medium heat.
2. Add sesame seeds, chili flakes, ginger, garlic, turmeric powder, and salt. Sauté for a couple of minutes.
3. Add broccoli and black beans and sauté until thoroughly heated. Sprinkle lime juice and serve hot.

Nutrition: Calories: 306 Carbs: 8g Fat: 16g Protein: 31g

17.   **Stuffed Peppers**

Preparation time: 15 minutes

Cooking time: 15 minutes

Servings: 8

Ingredients:

- 2 cans black beans, (15 oz), drained & rinsed
- 2 cups tofu, pressed, crumbled
- 3/4 cup green onion s, thinly sliced
- 1/2 cup fresh cilantro, chopped
- 1/4 cup vegetable oil
- 1/4 cup lime juice
- 3 cloves garlic, finely chopped
- 1/2 teaspoon salt
- 1/2 teaspoon chili powder
- 8 large bell peppers, halved lengthwise, deseeded
- 3 roma tomatoes, diced

Directions:

1. Mix in a bowl all the fixings except the bell peppers to make the filling. Fill the peppers with this mixture.
2. Cut 8 aluminum foils of size 18 x 12 inches. Place 2 halves on each aluminum foil. Seal the peppers such that there is a gap on the sides.

3. Grill under direct heat within 15 minutes. Sprinkle with some cilantro and serve.

Nutrition: Calories: 243 Carbs: 28g Fat: 7g Protein: 19g

18. Sweet 'N Spicy Tofu

Preparation time: 15 minutes

Cooking time: 30 minutes

Servings: 8

Ingredients:

- 14 ounces extra firm tofu; press the excess liquid and chop into cubes.
- 3 tablespoons olive oil
- 2 2-3 cloves garlic, minced
- 4 tablespoons sriracha sauce or any other hot sauce
- 2 tablespoons soy sauce
- 1/4 cup sweet chili sauce
- 5-6 cups mixed vegetables of your choice (like carrots, cauliflower, broccoli, potato, etc.)
- Salt to taste (optional)

Directions:

1. Place a nonstick pan over medium-high heat. Add 1 tablespoon oil. When oil is hot, add garlic and mixed vegetables and stir-fry until crisp and tender. Remove and keep aside.
2. Place the pan back on heat. Add 2 tablespoons oil. When oil is hot, add tofu and sauté until golden brown.

Add the sautéed vegetables. Mix well and remove from heat.

3. Make a mixture of sauces by mixing together all the sauces in a small bowl. Serve the stir-fried vegetables and tofu with sauce.

Nutrition: Calories: 270 Carbs: 41g Fat: 10g Protein: 12g

19. Eggplant & Mushrooms in Peanut Sauce

Preparation time: 15 minutes

Cooking time: 25 minutes

Servings: 6

Ingredients:

- 4 Japanese eggplants cut into 1-inch-thick round slices
- 3/4 pounds of shiitake mu shrooms, stems discarded, halved
- 3 tablespoons smooth peanut butter
- 2 1/2 tablespoons rice vinegar
- 1 1/2 tablespoons soy sauce
- 1 1/2 tablespoons, peeled, fresh ginger, finely grated
- 1 1/2 tablespoons light brown sugar
- Coarse salt to taste
- 3 scallions, cut into 2-inch lengths, thinly sliced lengthwise

Directions:

1. Place the eggplants and mushroom in a steamer. Steam the eggplant and mushrooms until tender. Transfer to a bowl. Put peanut butter and vinegar to a small bowl, and whisk.

2. Add rest of the fixings and whisk well. Add this to the bowl of eggplant slices. Add scallions and mix well. Serve hot.

Nutrition: Calories: 104 Carbs: 11g Fat: 6g Protein: 4g

20. Green Beans Stir Fry

Preparation time: 15 minutes

Cooking time: 15 minutes

Servings: 6-8

Ingredients:

- 1 1/2 pounds of green beans, stringed, chopped into 1 ½-inch pieces
- 1 large onion, thinly sliced
- 4-star anise (optional)
- 3 tablespoons avocado oil
- 1 1/2 tablespoons tamari sauce or soy sauce
- Salt to taste
- 3/4 cup water

Directions:

1. Place a wok over medium heat. Add oil. When oil is heated, add onions and sauté until onions are translucent.
2. Add beans, water, tamari sauce, and star anise and stir. Cover and cook until the beans are tender.
3. Uncover, add salt and raise the heat to high. Cook until the water dries up in the wok. Stir a couple of times while cooking.

Nutrition: Calories: 95 Carbs: 11g Fat: 5g Protein: 3g

21. **Dijon Maple Burgers**

Preparation Time: 20 minutes

Cooking Time: 30 minutes

Servings: 12

Ingredients:

- 1 red bell pepper
- 19 ounces can chickpeas, rinsed & drained
- 1 cup almonds, ground
- 2 teaspoons Dijon mustard
- 1 teaspoon oregano
- ½ teaspoon sage
- 1 cup spinach, fresh
- 1 – ½ cups rolled oats
- 1 clove garlic, pressed
- ½ lemon, juiced
- 2 teaspoons maple syrup, pure

Directions:

1. Get out a baking sheet. Line it with parchment paper. Cut your red pepper in half and then take the seeds out. Place it on your baking sheet, and roast in the oven while you prepare your other ingredients.

2. Process your chickpeas, almonds, mustard, and maple syrup together in a food processor. Add in your lemon

juice, oregano, sage, garlic, and spinach, processing again. Make sure it's combined, but don't puree it.

3. Once your red bell pepper is softened, which should roughly take ten minutes, add this to the processor as well. Add in your oats, mixing well.

4. Form twelve patties, cooking in the oven for a half-hour. They should be browned.

Nutrition: Calories: 96 Protein: 5.28 g Fat: 2.42 g Carbohydrates: 16.82 g

22. **Black Lentil Curry**

Preparation Time: 30 minutes

Cooking Time: 6 hours and 15 minutes

Servings: 4

Ingredients:

- 1 cup of black lentils, rinsed and soaked overnight
- 14 ounces of chopped tomatoes
- 2 large white onions, peeled and sliced
- 1 1/2 teaspoon of minced garlic
- 1 teaspoon of grated ginger
- 1 red chili
- 1 teaspoon of salt
- 1/4 teaspoon of red chili powder
- 1 teaspoon of paprika
- 1 teaspoon of ground turmeric
- 2 teaspoons of ground cumin
- 2 teaspoons of ground coriander
- 1/2 cup of chopped coriander
- 4-ounce of vegetarian butter
- 4 fluid of ounce water
- 2 fluid of ounce vegetarian double cream

Directions:

1. Place a large pan over moderate heat, add butter and let heat until melt. Add the onion and garlic and ginger and cook for 10 to 15 minutes or until onions are caramelized.
2. Then stir in salt, red chili powder, paprika, turmeric, cumin, ground coriander, and water. Transfer this mixture to a 6-quarts slow cooker and add tomatoes and red chili.
3. Drain lentils, add to slow cooker, and stir until just mix. Plugin slow cooker; adjust cooking time to 6 hours and let cook on low heat setting.
4. When the lentils are done, stir in cream and adjust the seasoning. Serve with boiled rice or whole wheat bread.

Nutrition: Calories: 299 Protein: 5.59 g Fat: 27.92 g Carbohydrates: 9.83 g

23. Flavorful Refried Beans

Preparation Time: 15 minutes

Cooking Time: 8 hours

Servings: 8

Ingredients:

- 3 cups of pinto beans, rinsed
- 1 small jalapeno pepper, seeded and chopped
- 1 medium-sized white onion, peeled and sliced
- 2 tablespoons of minced garlic
- 5 teaspoons of salt
- 2 teaspoons of ground black pepper
- 1/4 teaspoon of ground cumin
- 9 cups of water

Directions:

1. Using a 6-quarts slow cooker, place all the ingredients and stir until it mixes properly. Cover the top, plug in the slow cooker, adjust the cooking time to 6 hours, let it cook on the high heat setting, and add more water if the beans get too dry.

2. When the beans are done, drain it then reserve the liquid. Mash the beans using a potato masher and pour in the reserved cooking liquid until it reaches your desired mixture.

3. Serve immediately.

Nutrition: Calories: 268 Protein: 16.55 g Fat: 1.7 g Carbohydrates: 46.68 g

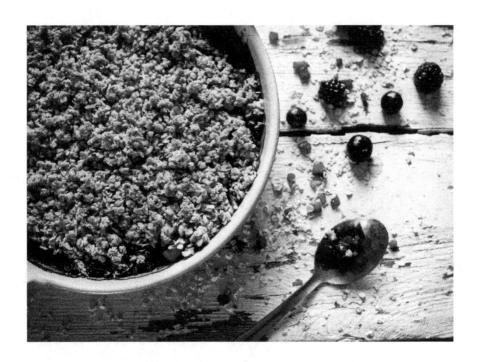

SNACKS

24. Mixed Seed Crackers

Preparation Time: 20 minutes

Cooking Time: 40 minutes

Servings: 30

Ingredients:

- 1 cup boiling water
- ¼ cup coconut oil, melted
- 1 tsp salt
- 1 tbsp. psyllium husk powder
- 1/3 cup of the following:
- Sesame seeds
- Flaxseed
- Pumpkin seeds, unsalted
- Sunflower seeds, unsalted
- Almond flour

Directions:

1. Set the oven to 300F. With a fork, combine the almond flour, seeds, psyllium, and salt. Cautiously pour the boiling water and oil to the bowl, using the fork to combine.

2. The mixture should form a gel-like consistency. Line a cookie sheet using a non-stick paper or a similar alternative, and transfer the mixture to the cookie sheet.

3. Using the second sheet of parchment, place it on top of the mixture, and with a rolling pin, roll out the mixture to an even and flat consistency.

4. Remove the top parchment paper then bake within 40 minutes, frequently checking to ensure the seeds do not burn.

5. After 40 minutes, or when the seeds are browning, turn off the oven but leave the crackers inside for further cooking. Once cool, break into pieces and enjoy.

Nutrition: Calories: 28 Protein: 0.44 g Fat: 2.15 g Carbohydrates: 1.89 g

25. **Crispy Squash Chips**

Preparation Time: 10 minutes

Cooking Time: 20 minutes

Servings: 2

Ingredients:

- 1 tsp cayenne pepper
- 1 tsp cumin
- 1 tsp paprika
- 1 tbsp. avocado oil
- 1 medium butternut squash, skinny neck
- Sea salt to taste

Directions:

1. Set the oven to 375 heat setting. Prepare the butternut squash by removing the top. Using a mandolin, cut the squash into even slices; it is unnecessary to skin the squash.
2. In a big mixing bowl, place your slices of squash and cover with oil, use your hands to mix them well. Ensure all slices are oiled.
3. Line a cookie sheet using parchment paper and spread out your slices, so they do not overlap.

4. In a little bowl, mix together cayenne pepper, paprika, and cumin, then sprinkle the chips over the top. Season with sea salt to taste. Once cool, enjoy alone or with your favorite dip.

Nutrition: Calories: 113 Protein: 3.66 g Fat: 10.57 g Carbohydrates: 1.6 g

26. Paprika Nuts

Preparation Time: 15 minutes

Cooking Time: 15 minutes

Servings: 8

Ingredients:

- 1 ½ tsp smoked paprika
- 1 tsp salt
- 2 tbsp. garlic-infused olive oil
- 1 cup of the following:
- Cashews
- Almonds
- Pecans
- Walnuts

Directions:

1. Adjust the rack in the middle of your oven. Set the oven to 325 before you start preparing the ingredients.
2. In a big mixing bowl, toss the nuts. Pour olive oil over the nuts and toss to coat all the nuts.
3. Sprinkle the salt and paprika over the nuts and mix well. If you want more paprika flavor, then add additional paprika.

4. Line a big cookie sheet using parchment and spread the nuts out in one layer. Bake for approximately 15 minutes, then remove from oven and let cool. Enjoy.

Nutrition: Calories: 67 Protein: 1.28 g Fat: 2.46 g Carbohydrates: 11.29 g

27. **Basil Zoodles and Olives**

Preparation Time: 30 minutes

Cooking Time: 4 hours

Servings: 6

Ingredients:

- 1 can black olives pitted
- 1 little container cherry tomatoes, halved
- 4 medium-size zucchinis
- Sauce:
- ½ cup basil leaves, chopped
- ½ tsp pink Himalayan salt
- 2 tsp nutritional yeast
- 1 tbsp. lemon juice
- ½ cup water
- ¼ cup of the following:
- Sunflower seeds, soaked
- Cashew nuts, soaked

Directions:

1. Begin by preparing the sunflower seeds and cashews. Place each in a little bowl and cover with water. Allow to soak for 4 hours, then drain and rinse well.

2. Next, place the seeds and cashews into a blender and mix until completely blended. Then add in basil, salt,

nutritional yeast, lemon juice, and water. Blend until a smooth sauce is formed.

3. Using a spiralizer, make the zoodles from the zucchini. Place the zoodles in a big serving bowl and then pour the sauce over the top. Stir to combine. Top with cherry tomatoes and olives. Serve and enjoy.

Nutrition: Calories: 56 Protein: 3.28 g Fat: 1.54 g Carbohydrates: 8.58 g

28. Roasted Beetroot Noodles

Preparation Time: 15 minutes

Cooking Time: 20 minutes

Servings: 4

Ingredients:

- 1 tsp orange zest
- 2 tbsp. of the following:
- Parsley, chopped
- Balsamic vinegar
- Olive oil
- 2 big beets, peeled and spiraled

Directions:

1. Set the oven to 425 high-heat settings. In a big bowl, combine the beet noodles, olive oil, and vinegar. Toss until well combined. Season with pepper and salt.
2. Line a big cookie sheet using parchment paper, and spread the noodles out into a single layer. Roast the noodles for 20 minutes.
3. Place into bowls and zest with orange and sprinkle parsley. Gently toss and serve.

Nutrition: Calories: 44 Protein: 2.71 g Fat: 1.71 g Carbohydrates: 5.02 g

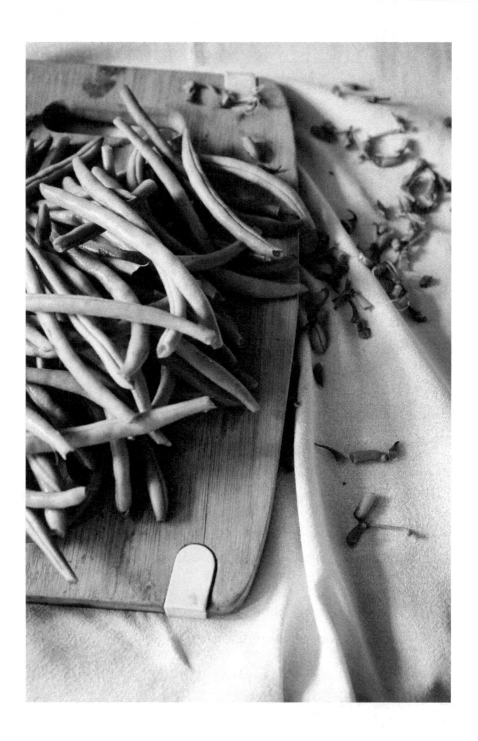

VEGETABLES

29. Sweet and Sour Tempeh

Preparation Time: 10 minutes

Cooking Time: 8 minutes

Serving: 4

Ingredient:

- 1 cup pineapple juice
- 1 tablespoon unseasoned rice vinegar
- 1 tablespoon soy sauce
- 1 tablespoon cornstarch
- 2 tablespoons coconut oil
- 1-pound tempeh, cut into thin strips
- 6 green onions
- 1 green bell pepper, diced
- 4 garlic cloves, minced
- 2 cups prepared brown or white rice

Direction

1. Blend pineapple juice, rice vinegar, soy sauce, and cornstarch and set aside.

2. In a wok or large sauté pan, heat the coconut oil over medium-high heat until it shimmers. Add the tempeh,

green onions, and bell pepper and cook until vegetables soften, about 5 minutes.

3. Cook garlic. Stir in sauce and cook until it thickens. Serve over rice.

Nutrition: 95 Calories 2g Fiber 5g Protein

30. **Fried Seitan Fingers**

Preparation Time: 15 minutes

Cooking Time: 10 minutes

Serving: 4

Ingredient:

- 1 cup all-purpose flour
- 1 teaspoon garlic powder
- 1 teaspoon onion powder
- Pinch of cayenne pepper
- 1 teaspoon dried thyme
- ½ teaspoon sea salt
- ½ teaspoon freshly ground black pepper
- 1 cup soy milk
- 1 tablespoon lemon juice
- 2 tablespoons baking powder
- 2 tablespoons olive oil
- 8 ounces Seitan

Direction

1. In a shallow dish, incorporate flour, garlic powder, onion powder, cayenne, thyme, salt, and black pepper, whisking to mix thoroughly. In another shallow dish, whisk together the soy milk, lemon juice, and baking powder.

2. In sauté pan, cook the olive oil over medium-high heat. Dip each piece of seitan in the flour mixture, tapping off any excess flour. Next, dip the seitan in the soy milk mixture and then back in the flour mixture.

3. Fry for 4 minutes per side. Blot on paper towels before serving.

Nutrition: 100 Calories 4g Fiber 8g Protein

SALAD

31.   Lentil Radish Salad

Preparation Time: 15 minutes

Cooking Time: 0 minutes

Servings: 3

Ingredients:

- Dressing:
- 1 tbsp. extra virgin olive oil
- 1 tbsp. lemon juice
- 1 tbsp. maple syrup
- 1 tbsp. water
- ½ tbsp. sesame oil
- 1 tbsp. miso paste, yellow or white
- ¼ tsp. salt
- ¼ tsp Pepper
- Salad:
- ½ cup dry chickpeas
- ¼ cup dry green or brown lentils
- 1 14-oz. pack of silken tofu
- 5 cups mixed greens, fresh or frozen
- 2 radishes, thinly sliced

- ½ cup cherry tomatoes, halved
- ¼ cup roasted sesame seeds

Directions:

1. Prepare the chickpeas according to the method.
2. Prepare the lentils according to the method.
3. Put all the ingredients for the dressing in a blender or food processor. Mix on low until smooth, while adding water until it reaches the desired consistency.
4. Add salt, pepper (to taste), and optionally more water to the dressing; set aside.
5. Cut the tofu into bite-sized cubes.
6. Combine the mixed greens, tofu, lentils, chickpeas, radishes, and tomatoes in a large bowl.
7. Add the dressing and mix everything until it is coated evenly.
8. Top with the optional roasted sesame seeds, if desired.
9. Refrigerate before serving and enjoy, or, store for later!

Nutrition: Calories 621 Total Fat 19.6g Saturated Fat 2.8g Cholesterol 0mg Sodium 996mg Total Carbohydrate 82.7g Dietary Fiber 26.1g Total Sugars 20.7g Protein 31.3g Vitamin D 0mcg Calcium 289mg Iron 9mg Potassium 1370mg

GRAINS

32. Vegetable and Wild Rice Pilaf

Preparation Time: 10 minutes

Cooking Time: 48 to 49 minutes

Servings: 6

Ingredients:

- 1 potato, scrubbed and chopped
- 1 cup chopped cauliflower
- 1 cup chopped scallion
- 1 cup chopped broccoli
- 1 to 2 cloves garlic, minced
- 2 tablespoons soy sauce
- 3 cups low-sodium vegetable broth
- 1 cup long-grain brown rice
- 1/3 cup wild rice
- 2 small zucchinis, chopped
- ½ cup grated carrot
- 1/8 teaspoon sesame oil (optional)
- ¼ cup chopped fresh cilantro
- ½ cup water

Directions:

1. Bring the water to a boil in a large saucepan. Add the potato, cauliflower, scallion, broccoli and garlic and sauté for 2 to 3 minutes.

2. Add the soy sauce and cook for 1 minute. Add the vegetable broth, brown rice and wild rice. Bring to a boil. Reduce the heat, cover, and cook for 15 minutes.

3. Stir in the zucchinis. After another 15 minutes, stir in the carrot. Continue to cook for 15 minutes. Stir in the sesame oil (if desired) and cilantro.

4. Serve immediately.

Nutrition: calories: 376 fat: 3.6g carbs: 74.5g protein: 11.8g fiber: 8.1g

33. Brown Rice with Spiced Vegetables

Preparation Time: 10 minutes

Cooking Time: 16 to 18 minutes

Servings: 6

Ingredients:

- 2 teaspoons grated fresh ginger
- 2 cloves garlic, crushed
- ½ cup water
- ¼ pound (113 g) green beans, trimmed and cut into 1-inch pieces
- 1 carrot, scrubbed and sliced
- ½ pound (227 g) mushrooms, sliced
- 2 zucchinis, cut in half lengthwise and sliced
- 1 bunch scallions, cut into 1-inch pieces
- 4 cups cooked brown rice
- 3 tablespoons soy sauce

Directions:

1. Place the ginger and garlic in a large pot with the water. Add the green beans and carrot and sauté for 3 minutes.
2. Add the mushrooms and sauté for another 2 minutes. Stir in the zucchini and scallions. Reduce the heat.

Cover and cook for 6 to 8 minutes, or until the vegetables are tender-crisp, stirring frequently.

3. Stir in the rice and soy sauce. Cook over low heat for 5 minutes, or until heated through.

4. Serve warm.

Nutrition: calories: 205 fat: 3.0g carbs: 38.0g protein: 6.4g fiber:4.4 g

34. <u>Spiced Tomato Brown Rice</u>

Preparation Time: 10 minutes

Cooking Time: 15 minutes

Servings: 4 to 6

Ingredients:

- 1 onion, diced
- 1 green bell pepper, diced
- 3 cloves garlic, minced
- ¼ cup water
- 15 to 16 ounces (425 to 454g) tomatoes, chopped
- 1 tablespoon chili powder
- 2 teaspoons ground cumin
- 1 teaspoon dried basil
- ½ teaspoon Parsley Patch seasoning, general blend
- ¼ teaspoon cayenne
- 2 cups cooked brown rice

Directions:

1. Combine the onion, green pepper, garlic and water in a saucepan over medium heat. Cook for about 5 minutes, stirring constantly, or until softened.

2. Add the tomatoes and seasonings. Cook for another 5 minutes. Stir in the cooked rice. Cook for another 5 minutes to allow the flavors to blend.

3. Serve immediately.

Nutrition: calories: 107 fat: 1.1g carbs: 21.1g protein: 3.2g fiber: 2.9g

LEGUMES

35. Indian Dal Makhani

Preparation Time: 10 minutes

Cooking Time: 10 minutes

Servings: 4

Ingredients:

- 3 tablespoons sesame oil
- 1 large onion, chopped
- 1 bell pepper, seeded and chopped
- 2 garlic cloves, minced
- 1 tablespoon ginger, grated
- 2 green chilies, seeded and chopped
- 1 teaspoon cumin seeds
- 1 bay laurel
- 1 teaspoon turmeric powder
- 1/4 teaspoon red peppers
- 1/4 teaspoon ground allspice
- 1/2 teaspoon garam masala
- 1 cup tomato sauce
- 4 cups vegetable broth
- 1 ½ cups black lentils, soaked overnight and drained

- 4-5 curry leaves, for garnish

Directions

1. In a saucepan, heat the sesame oil over medium-high heat; now, sauté the onion and bell pepper for 3 minutes more until they've softened.

2. Add in the garlic, ginger, green chilies, cumin seeds and bay laurel; continue to sauté, stirring frequently, for 1 minute or until fragrant.

3. Stir in the remaining ingredients, except for the curry leaves. Now, turn the heat to a simmer. Continue to cook for 15 minutes more or until thoroughly cooked.

4. Garnish with curry leaves and serve hot!

Nutrition: Calories: 329; Fat: 8.5g; Carbs: 44.1g; Protein: 16.8g

36. **Mexican-Style Bean Bowl**

Preparation Time: 10 minutes

Cooking Time: 10 minutes

Servings: 4

Ingredients:

- 1-pound red beans, soaked overnight and drained
- 1 cup canned corn kernels, drained
- 2 roasted bell peppers, sliced
- 1 chili pepper, finely chopped
- 1 cup cherry tomatoes, halved
- 1 red onion, chopped
- 1/4 cup fresh cilantro, chopped
- 1/4 cup fresh parsley, chopped
- 1 teaspoon Mexican oregano
- 1/4 cup red wine vinegar
- 2 tablespoons fresh lemon juice
- 1/3 cup extra-virgin olive oil
- Sea salt and ground black, to taste
- 1 avocado, peeled, pitted and sliced

Directions

1. Cover the soaked beans with a fresh change of cold water and bring to a boil. Let it boil for about 10

minutes. Turn the heat to a simmer and continue to cook for 50 to 55 minutes or until tender.

2. Allow your beans to cool completely, then, transfer them to a salad bowl.

3. Add in the remaining ingredients and toss to combine well. Serve at room temperature.

4. Bon appétit!

Nutrition: Calories: 465; Fat: 17.9g; Carbs: 60.4g; Protein: 20.2g

BREAD & PIZZA

37. Spinach Cheese Flatbread Pizza

Preparation time: 10 minutes

Cooking time: 20 minutes

Servings: 3

Ingredients:

- Garlic naan flatbread – 1
- Crushed red pepper flakes – 1/8 teaspoon.
- Pesto – 2 teaspoons.
- Feta cheese – 2 tablespoons, crumbled
- Mozzarella cheese – 2 oz., grated
- Parmesan cheese – 1/4 cup, grated
- Heavy cream – 1/4 cup
- Garlic clove – 1, minced
- Butter – 1 tablespoon.
- Fresh spinach – 5 oz., chopped
- Salt – 1/8 teaspoon.

Directions:

1. Preheat the oven to 350 F. Melt butter in a deep pan over medium-high heat.

2. Add spinach and garlic and sauté until spinach is wilted. Add parmesan cheese, heavy cream, and salt and turn heat to low and simmer until thickened, about 5 minutes.
3. Stir frequently. Remove pan from heat and allow to cool. Spread spinach mixture on flatbread and top with feta cheese and mozzarella cheese.
4. Drizzle with pesto and bake in a preheated oven for 12 minutes. Serve.

Nutrition: Calories: 250 Cal, Carbohydrates: 25g, Protein: 5g, Fats: 8g, Fiber: 1g.

38. **Fluffy Deep-Dish Pizza**

Preparation time: 10 minutes

Cooking time: 2 hours

Servings: 6

Ingredients:

- 12 inch of frozen whole-wheat pizza crust, thawed
- 1 medium-sized red bell pepper, cored and sliced
- 5-ounce of spinach leaves, chopped
- 1 small red onion, peeled and chopped
- 1 1/2 teaspoons of minced garlic
- 1/4 teaspoon of salt
- 1/2 teaspoon of red pepper flakes
- 1/2 teaspoon of dried thyme
- 1/4 cup of chopped basil, fresh
- 14-ounce of pizza sauce
- 1 cup of shredded vegan mozzarella

Directions:

1. Place a medium-sized non-stick skillet pan over an average heat, add the oil and let it heat.
2. Add the onion, garlic and let it cook for 5 minutes or until it gets soft.
3. Then add the red bell pepper and continue cooking for 4 minutes or until it becomes tender-crisp.

4. Add the spinach, salt, red pepper, thyme, basil and stir properly.

5. Cool off for 3 to 5 minutes or until the spinach leaves wilts, and then set it aside until it is called for.

6. Grease a 4-quarts slow cooker with a non-stick cooking spray and insert the pizza crust in it.

7. Press the dough into the bottom and spread 1 inch up along the sides.

8. Spread it with the pizza sauce, cover it with the spinach mixture and then garnish evenly with the cheese.

9. Sprinkle it with the red pepper flakes, basil leaves and cover it with the lid.

10. Plug in the slow cooker and let it cook for 1 1/2 hours to 2 hours at the low heat setting or until the crust turns golden brown and the cheese melts completely.

11. When done, transfer the pizza into the cutting board, let it rest for 10 minutes, then slice to serve.

Nutrition: Calories: 250 Cal, Carbohydrates: 25g, Protein: 5g, Fats: 8g, Fiber: 1g.

SOUP AND STEW

39. Broccoli Fennel Soup

Preparation Time: 15 Minutes

Cooking Time: 10 Minutes

Servings: 4

Ingredients:

- 1 fennel bulb, white and green parts coarsely chopped
- 10 oz. broccoli, cut into florets
- 3 cups vegetable stock
- Salt and freshly ground black pepper
- 1 garlic clove
- 1 cup dairy-free cream cheese
- 3 oz. vegan butter
- ½ cup chopped fresh oregano

Directions:

1. In a medium pot, combine the fennel, broccoli, vegetable stock, salt, and black pepper. Bring to a boil until the vegetables soften, 10 to 15 minutes.
2. Stir in the remaining ingredients and simmer the soup for 3 to 5 minutes.

3. Adjust the taste with salt and black pepper, and dish the soup.

4. Serve warm.

Nutrition: Calories 240 Fat 0 g Protein 0 g Carbohydrates 20 g

40. Tofu Goulash Soup

Preparation Time: 35 Minutes

Cooking Time: 20 Minutes

Servings: 4

Ingredients:

- 4¼ oz. vegan butter
- 1 white onion, chopped
- 2 garlic cloves, minced
- 1 ½ cups butternut squash
- 1 red bell pepper, deseeded and chopped
- 1 tbsp paprika powder
- ¼ tsp red chili flakes
- 1 tbsp dried basil
- ½ tbsp crushed cardamom seeds
- Salt and black pepper to taste
- 1 ½ cups crushed tomatoes
- 3 cups vegetable broth
- 1½ tsp red wine vinegar
- Chopped parsley to serve

Directions:

1. Place the tofu between two paper towels and allow draining of water for 30 minutes. After, crumble the tofu and set aside.

2. Melt the vegan butter in a large pot over medium heat and sauté the onion and garlic until the veggies are fragrant and soft, 3 minutes.

3. Stir in the tofu and cook until golden brown, 3 minutes.

4. Add the butternut squash, bell pepper, paprika, red chili flakes, basil, cardamom seeds, salt, and black pepper. Cook for 2 minutes to release some flavor and mix in the tomatoes and 2 cups of vegetable broth.

5. Close the lid, bring the soup to a boil, and then simmer for 10 minutes.

6. Stir in the remaining vegetable broth, the red wine vinegar, and adjust the taste with salt and black pepper.

7. Dish the soup, garnish with the parsley and serve warm.

Nutrition: Calories 320 Fat 10 g Protein 10 g Carbohydrates 20 g

SAUCES, DRESSINGS & DIP

41. Garlic White Bean Dip

Preparation Time: 15 minutes

Cooking Time: 15 minutes

Servings: 2

Ingredients:

- 1/4 cup soft bread crumbs
- 2 tablespoon dry white wine or water
- 2 tablespoons olive oil
- 2 tablespoon lemon juice
- 4-1/2 teaspoon. minced fresh parsley
- 3 garlic cloves, peeled and halved
- 1/2 teaspoon salt
- 1/2 teaspoon snipped fresh dill or 1/4 teaspoon dill weed
- 1/8 teaspoon cayenne pepper
- Assorted fresh vegetables

Directions:

1. Mix wine and bread crumbs in a small bowl. Mix cayenne, dill, salt, garlic, parsley, beans, lemon juice,

and oil in a food processor, then cover and blend until smooth.

2. Put in bread crumb mixture and process until well combined. Serve together with vegetables.

Nutrition: calories 105 fat 5 carbs 12 protein 6

42. **Fruit Skewers**

Preparation Time: 20 minutes

Cooking Time: 20 minutes

Servings: 2

Ingredients:

- cream cheese
- fat sour cream
- lime juice
- honey
- 1/2 teaspoon ground ginger
- 2 cups green grapes
- 2 cups fresh or canned unsweetened pineapple chunks
- 2 large red apples, cut into 1-inch pieces

Directions:

1. To make the dip, beat the sour cream and cream cheese in a small bowl until it becomes smooth. Beat in the ginger, honey, and lime juice until it becomes smooth.
2. Put the cover and let it chill in the fridge for a minimum of 1 hour.
3. Alternately thread the apples, pineapple, and grapes on 8 12-inch skewers. Serve it right away with the dip.

Nutrition: calories 180 fat 5 carbs 28 protein 4

43. Low-fat Stuffed Mushrooms

Preparation Time: 20 minutes

Cooking Time: 25 minutes

Servings: 6

Ingredients:

- 1 lb. large fresh mushrooms
- 3 tablespoons seasoned bread crumbs
- 3 tablespoons fat-free sour cream
- 2 tablespoons grated Parmesan cheese
- 2 tablespoons minced chives
- 2 tablespoons reduced-fat mayonnaise
- 2 teaspoons balsamic vinegar
- 2 to 3 drops hot pepper sauce, optional

Directions:

1. Take out the stems from the mushrooms, then put the cups aside. Chop the stems and set aside 1/3 cup (eliminate the leftover stems or reserve for later use).
2. Mix the reserved mushroom stems, hot pepper sauce if preferred, vinegar, mayonnaise, chives, Parmesan cheese, sour cream, and breadcrumbs in a bowl, then stir well.
3. Put the mushroom caps on a cooking spray-coated baking tray and stuff it with the crumb mixture.

4. Let it boil for 5 to 7 minutes, placed 4-6 inches from the heat source, or until it turns light brown.

Nutrition: calories 435 fat 4 carbs 23 protein 9

APPETIZER

44. **<u>Vegetable Medley</u>**

Preparation Time: 20 minutes

Cooking Time: 15 minutes

Servings: 1

Ingredients:

- 1 Tomato (diced)
- 1 pinch Garlic pepper seasoning
- 2 Fresh mushrooms (sliced)
- 2 Yellow squash (cubed)
- Cooking spray
- 2 Zucchini (cubed)

Directions:

1. Start by taking a large skillet and greasing it using the cooking spray. Place the skillet over medium flame and add in the tomatoes.
2. Let the tomatoes cook for about 5 minutes. Add in the garlic pepper seasoning. Toss in the mushrooms, zucchini and squash. Let them cook on a medium flame for about 15 minutes. Serve.

Nutrition: Calories: 49 Carbs: 1g Fat: 5g Protein: 0g

45. White Beans with Collard Greens

Preparation Time: 15 minutes

Cooking Time: 40 minutes

Servings: 1

Ingredients

- 2 tbsp Water
- 1 ¼ cup Onion (chopped)
- 3 tbsp Garlic (minced)
- 1 cube Vegetarian bouillon (beef-flavored)
- 7 oz Collard greens (chopped
- 14 ½ oz Diced tomatoes, no added salt (1 can)
- 1 ¼ cup Water
- Salt, as per taste
- Black pepper (freshly ground), as per taste
- 14 ½ oz Great Northern beans (1 can)
- 1 tsp White sugar

Directions:

1. Start by placing a large nonstick skillet on medium flame. Pour in 2 tablespoons of water. Let it heat through.

2. Stir in garlic and onion and cook for about 10 minutes. Add in more water if required to avoid scorching. Add in the vegetarian bouillon to the pan. Keep stirring.

3. Toss in the collard greens and tomatoes to the onion mixture. Also add in 1 ¼ cups of water.

4. Season the mixture with pepper and salt. Cover with a lid and cook for about 20 minutes. Make sure that all vegetables become tender.

5. Now add in the sugar and beans and cook for about 10 minutes. Serve.

Nutrition: Calories: 251 Carbs: 39g Fat: 3g Protein: 19g

SMOOTHIES AND JUICES

46. Pumpkin Smoothie

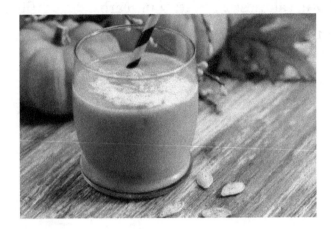

Preparation Time: 5 minutes

Cooking Time: 0 minutes

Servings: 5

Ingredients:

- ½ cup pumpkin purée
- 4 Medjool dates, pitted and chopped
- 1 cup unsweetened almond milk
- ¼ teaspoon vanilla extract
- ¼ teaspoon ground cinnamon
- ½ cup ice
- Pinch ground nutmeg

Directions:

1. Add all the ingredients in a blender, then process until the mixture is glossy and well mixed.
2. Serve immediately.

Nutrition: calories: 417 fat: 3.0g carbs: 94.9g fiber: 10.4g protein: 11.4g

47. **Super Smoothie**

Preparation Time: 5 minutes

Cooking Time: 0 minutes

Servings: 4

Ingredients:

- 1 banana, peeled
- 1 cup chopped mango
- 1 cup raspberries
- ¼ cup rolled oats
- 1 carrot, peeled
- 1 cup chopped fresh kale
- 2 tablespoons chopped fresh parsley
- 1 tablespoon flaxseeds
- 1 tablespoon grated fresh ginger
- ½ cup unsweetened soy milk
- 1 cup water

Directions:

1. Put all the ingredients in a food processor, then blitz until glossy and smooth.
2. Serve immediately or chill in the refrigerator for an hour before serving.

Nutrition: calories: 550 fat: 39.0g carbs: 31.0g fiber: 15.0g protein: 13.0g

DESERTS

48. Cookie Dough

Preparation time: 25 minutes

Cooking time: 0 minutes

Servings: 18-20

Ingredients:

- 8 tablespoons unsalted grass-fed butter, at room temperature
- 1/3 cup Swerve sweetener
- ½ teaspoon vanilla extract
- ¼ teaspoon salt
- 2 cups almond flour
- ½ cup dark chocolate chips

Directions:

1. In the bowl of a stand mixer, combine the butter, Swerve, vanilla, and salt. Beat until the mixture is light and fluffy.
2. Add the almond flour and continue to mix on low until a dough form. Fold in the chocolate chips until just barely combined.

3. Place the dough in refrigerator for about 15 minutes to set. Line a baking sheet with parchment paper.

4. Using a 2-inch cookie scoop, scoop balls of dough onto the prepared baking sheet. Store the cookie-dough balls in the refrigerator until ready to eat.

Nutrition: Calories: 122 Fat: 10g Protein: 2g Carbs: 6g

49. No-Bake Coconut Cookies

Preparation time: 40 minutes

Cooking time: 5 minutes

Servings: 12

Ingredients:

- 2 tablespoons grass-fed butter
- 2/3 cup crunchy natural peanut butter
- 1½ tablespoons unsweetened cocoa powder
- 5 or 6 drops liquid stevia
- 1 cup finely shredded unsweetened coconut flakes

Directions:

1. Line a baking sheet with parchment paper. Dissolve the butter in a medium saucepan over medium heat. Add the peanut butter and cocoa powder, and stir well.
2. Remove from the heat and add the stevia. Stir in the coconut flakes and mix until all the ingredients are well combined.
3. Scoop the dough in small spoonful onto the prepared baking sheet. Put the baking sheet in the refrigerator within 30 minutes to set. Serve.

Nutrition: Calories: 153 Fat: 13g Protein: 4g Carbs: 5g

50. __Lemon Bars__

Preparation time: 15 minutes

Cooking time: 25 minutes

Servings: 9

Ingredients:

- Nonstick cooking spray
- 1 1/8 cups almond flour
- 1/8 cup powdered erythritol sweetener, plus 2/3 cup, plus more for sprinkling
- 1/3 cup coconut oil, melted
- 2 large organic eggs
- 2 tablespoons + 2 teaspoons freshly squeezed lemon juice
- ¼ teaspoon baking powder
- ½ tablespoon coconut flour

Directions:

1. Preheat the oven to 350°F. Spray an 8-by-8-inch baking dish with cooking spray. In a small bowl, combine the almond flour and 1/8 cup of erythritol. Add the melted coconut oil and blend until the mixture is crumbly.

2. Put the crust batter to press into the bottom of the prepared baking dish. Bake within 10 minutes, or until the crust is slightly golden brown.

3. In a high-powered blender, combine the eggs, remaining 2/3 cup of erythritol, lemon juice, baking powder, and coconut flour, and blend for about 30 seconds.

4. Put the filling into the crust and cook for an additional 10 to 12 minutes, or until the filling is set. Remove from the oven and sprinkle with a dusting of powdered sweetener. Allow to cool, then serve.

Nutrition: Calories: 128 Fat: 12g Protein: 3g Carbs: 2g

51. __Peanut Butter Cookies__

Preparation time: 10 minutes

Cooking time: 10 minutes

Servings: 12

Ingredients:

- Nonstick cooking spray
- 1 cup chunky natural peanut butter
- ¾ cup erythritol, granulated
- 1 organic egg, beaten

Directions:

1. Preheat the oven to 350°F. Spray a baking sheet with cooking spray. Combine the peanut butter and erythritol in a medium mixing bowl. Mix well.
2. Add the egg and stir until thoroughly combined. Using a 2-inch cookie scoop, roll the dough into balls and set them on the prepared baking sheet.
3. Using the back of a fork, press a crisscross pattern onto the top of each cookie. Bake for 9 to 10 minutes, then transfer to a wire rack to cool.

Nutrition: Calories: 135 Fat: 11g Protein: 5g Carbs: 4g

52. Fudge Brownies

Preparation time: 15 minutes

Cooking time: 20 minutes

Servings: 12

Ingredients:

- Nonstick cooking spray
- 12 tablespoons (1½ sticks) grass-fed butter
- 2 ounces dark chocolate squares (80 percent or higher), broken into chunks
- ¼ cup unsweetened cocoa powder
- ½ cup almond flour
- 2/3 cup Swerve sweetener
- ½ teaspoon baking powder
- 3 large organic eggs, beaten

Directions:

1. Warm your oven to 350°F. Oiled an 8-by-8-inch baking dish with cooking spray. In a small saucepan over low heat, melt the butter and dark chocolate while stirring.

2. When melted, add the cocoa powder and stir until combined. Set aside. In a small mixing bowl, combine the almond flour, Swerve, and baking powder. Stir well.

3. In a separate bowl, pour in the eggs and then slowly stir in the dark chocolate mixture. Mix together for

about 1 minute to make sure everything is well combined.

4. Pour the flour mixture into the chocolate mixture and stir until a batter form. Spread the batter into the prepared baking dish and cook for 18 to 20 minutes, or until a toothpick inserted into the center comes out clean.

5. Remove then allow to cool before cutting into 12 squares.

Nutrition: Calories: 163 Fat: 15g Protein: 3g Carbs: 4g

CPSIA information can be obtained
at www.ICGtesting.com
Printed in the USA
LVHW061642200421
685034LV00011B/713

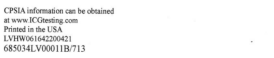

9 781801 832953